IMG Friendly Physical Medicine and
Rehabilitation PM&R Residency Programs List
With Comprehensive Match Selection Criteria
and Programs Requirements

By

IMG Guide

And

Applicant Guide

Introduction

IMG Friendly Physical Medicine and Rehabilitation Residency Programs

In Collaboration between the Applicant Guide and the IMG Guide we present to you the most complete and up-to-date IMG friendly Physical Medicine and Rehabilitation PM&R residency programs list with full match selection criteria and requirements for these programs. This book is essentially written for international medical graduates seeking residency in the US. The idea of writing this book came from our insight that many IMGs every year don't match because they don't know where to apply. Most of the time, they end applying to programs that don't have IMGs or those that don't match their criteria hence they end losing money with no interviews earned. The information was gathered from program directors, coordinators, chiefs, faculty and residents. It includes Programs names, Programs codes, States, Addresses, Phones, Faxes, Percentage of IMGs in the programs, Minimum USMLE Step 1 and Step 2 Score Requirements, Attempts on any step, CS requirement at time of application, USCE Requirements, Cut-Off time since graduation, Programs offering couple match and Visas Sponsored or accepted.

Disclaimer: We are not affiliated to any official or non official organization. We are not affiliated to ECFMG, ERAS, NRMP or USMLE.

Disclaimer: The information in this book is personally collected by the author from various resources in the residency programs which is/are subject to change by/at the programs at any time. Although we did our best to get the most accurate information as much as possible from the program directors, coordinators, faculty and residents, however, you understand that by reading this book you are using the information here on your own responsibility.

Arkansas

University of Arkansas for Medical Sciences Physical Medicine and Rehabilitation Residency Program

Specialty: Physical Medicine and Rehabilitation

Program name: University of Arkansas for Medical Sciences Program
Program code: 340-04-21-083
State: Arkansas
Address: University of Arkansas for Medical Sciences
4301 W Markham St, Little Rock, AR 72205
Phone: (501) 526-7732
Percentage of IMGs in the program: 20%
Minimum USMLE Step 1 Score Requirement: No limits set
Minimum USMLE Step 2 Score Requirement: No limits set
Attempts on any step: No limits set
CS required at time of application: Yes
USCE Requirement: None
Cut-Off time since graduation: No limits set
Program offers couple match: Yes
Visas Sponsored or accepted: J1 visa

California

Loma Linda University Physical Medicine and Rehabilitation Residency Program

Specialty: Physical Medicine and Rehabilitation

Program name: Loma Linda University Program
Program code: 340-05-21-077
NRMP Code: 1024340C0
Program type: University-based
State: California
Address: Loma Linda University Medical Center
11406 Loma Linda Dr, Loma Linda, CA 92354
Phone: (909) 558-6204
Fax: (909) 558-6110
Percentage of IMGs in the program: 15%
Minimum USMLE Step 1 Score Requirement: 215
Minimum USMLE Step 2 Score Requirement: 215
Attempts on any step: Must pass on first attempt on any step
CS required at time of application: Yes including ECFMG certificate and PTAL/Status letter
USCE Requirement: None
Cut-Off time since graduation: No limits set
Program offers couple match: Yes
Visas Sponsored or accepted: J1 visa

Stanford University Physical Medicine and Rehabilitation Residency Program

Specialty: Physical Medicine and Rehabilitation

Program name: Stanford University Program
Program code: 340-05-21-008
State: California
Address: Stanford Medicine Outpatient Center
450 Broadway St, Redwood City, CA 94063
Phone: (650) 721-7627
Fax: (650) 721-3470
Percentage of IMGs in the program: 5%
Minimum USMLE Step 1 Score Requirement: 220
Minimum USMLE Step 2 Score Requirement: 220
Attempts on any step: Must pass on first attempt on any step
CS required at time of application: Yes including ECFMG certificate and PTAL/Status letter
USCE Requirement: None
Cut-Off time since graduation: No limits set
Program offers couple match: Yes
Visas Sponsored or accepted: J1 visa

VA Greater Los Angeles Healthcare System Physical Medicine and Rehabilitation Residency Program

Specialty: Physical Medicine and Rehabilitation
Program name: VA Greater Los Angeles Healthcare System Program

Program code: 340-05-21-007
NRMP Code: 1039340A0
Program type: Community-based university affiliated hospital
State: California
Address: VA Greater Los Angeles Healthcare System

11301 Wilshire Blvd, Los Angeles, CA 90073
Phone: (310) 268-3342
Fax: (310) 268-4224
Percentage of IMGs in the program: 10%
Minimum USMLE Step 1 Score Requirement: No limits set
Minimum USMLE Step 2 Score Requirement: No limits set
Attempts on any step: No limits set
CS required at time of application: No but PTAL/Status letter required
USCE Requirement: Yes 4 months
Cut-Off time since graduation: No limits set
Program offers couple match: Yes
Visas Sponsored or accepted: J1 visa

University of California (Irvine) Physical Medicine and Rehabilitation Residency Program

Specialty: Physical Medicine and Rehabilitation

Program name: University of California (Irvine) Program
Program code: 340-05-21-005
State: California
Address: UC Irvine Medical Center
101 The City Dr S, Orange, CA 92868
Phone: (714) 456-6444
Fax: (714) 456-6557
Percentage of IMGs in the program: 15%
Minimum USMLE Step 1 Score Requirement: 205
Minimum USMLE Step 2 Score Requirement: 205
Attempts on any step: Must pass on first attempt including The CS exam
CS required at time of application: Yes including ECFMG certificate and PTAL/Status letter
USCE Requirement: Yes
Cut-Off time since graduation: No limits set
Program offers couple match: Yes
Visas Sponsored or accepted: J1 visa

District of Columbia

National Rehabilitation Hospital/Washington Hospital Center/Georgetown University Hospital Physical Medicine and Rehabilitation Residency Program

Specialty: Physical Medicine and Rehabilitation
Program name: National Rehabilitation Hospital/Washington Hospital Center/Georgetown University Hospital Program
Program code: 340-10-21-087
NRMP Code: 3191340A0
Program type: University-based
State: District of Columbia
Address: MedStar National Rehabilitation Hospital
102 Irving St NW, Washington, DC 20010
Phone: (202) 877-1627
Fax: (202) 877-1166
Percentage of IMGs in the program: 100%
Minimum USMLE Step 1 Score Requirement: No limits set
Minimum USMLE Step 2 Score Requirement: No limits set
Attempts on any step: No limits set
CS required at time of application: No
USCE Requirement: Yes
Cut-Off time since graduation: No limits set

Program offers couple match: Yes
Visas Sponsored or accepted: J1 visa

Florida

Jackson Memorial Hospital/Jackson Health System Physical Medicine and Rehabilitation Residency Program

Specialty: Physical Medicine and Rehabilitation
Program name: Jackson Memorial Hospital/Jackson Health System Program
Program code: 340-11-21-107
NRMP Code: 1104340A0
Program type: University-based
State: Florida
Address: University of Miami/Jackson Memorial Hospital
        1611 NW 12th Ave, Miami, FL 33136
Phone: (305) 585-1431
Fax: (305) 355-2424
Percentage of IMGs in the program: 20%

Minimum USMLE Step 1 Score Requirement: No limits set
Minimum USMLE Step 2 Score Requirement: No limits set
Attempts on any step: No limits set
CS required at time of application: No
USCE Requirement: None
Cut-Off time since graduation: No limits set
Program offers couple match: Yes
Visas Sponsored or accepted: J1 visa

University of South Florida Morsani (James A Haley Veterans Hospital) Physical Medicine and Rehabilitation Residency Program

Specialty: Physical Medicine and Rehabilitation
Program name: University of South Florida Morsani (James A Haley Veterans Hospital) Program
Program code: 340-11-13-106
State: Florida
Address: James A Haley Veterans Hospital
          13000 Bruce B Downs Blvd, Tampa, FL 33612
Phone: (813) 972-7688
Fax: (813) 903-2483
Percentage of IMGs in the program: 25%
Minimum USMLE Step 1 Score Requirement: No limits set

Minimum USMLE Step 2 Score Requirement:
No limits set
Attempts on any step: No limits set
CS required at time of application: Yes
USCE Requirement: Yes, 1 month
Cut-Off time since graduation: 5 years but must
be clinically active, otherwise 2 years.
Program offers couple match: Yes
Visas Sponsored or accepted: J1 visa

Georgia

Emory University Physical Medicine and Rehabilitation Residency Program

Specialty: Physical Medicine and Rehabilitation
Program name: Emory University Program
Program code: 340-12-21-011
State: Georgia
Address: Emory University School of Medicine
1441 Clifton Rd NE, Atlanta, GA 30322
Phone: (404) 712-5511
Fax: (404) 778-8358
Percentage of IMGs in the program: 10%
Minimum USMLE Step 1 Score Requirement:
No limits set

Minimum USMLE Step 2 Score Requirement: No limits set
Attempts on any step: No limits set
CS required at time of application: Yes including ECFMG certificate
USCE Requirement: None
Cut-Off time since graduation: No limits set
Program offers couple match: Yes
Visas Sponsored or accepted: J1 visa and H1b visa

Illinois

Loyola University Physical Medicine and Rehabilitation Residency Program

Specialty: Physical Medicine and Rehabilitation
Program name: Loyola University Program
Program code: 340-16-31-016
NRMP Code: 1170340A0
Program type: University-based
State: Illinois
Address: Loyola University Medical Center
2160 S First Ave, Maywood, IL 60153
Phone: (708) 216-4254
Fax: (708) 216-9348

Percentage of IMGs in the program: 0% (occasionally one)
Minimum USMLE Step 1 Score Requirement: No limits set
Minimum USMLE Step 2 Score Requirement: No limits set
Attempts on any step: No limits set
CS required at time of application: No
USCE Requirement: Yes
Cut-Off time since graduation: 2 years
Program offers couple match: Yes
Visas Sponsored or accepted: J1 visa

Schwab Rehabilitation Hospital and Care Network/University of Chicago Physical Medicine and Rehabilitation Residency Program

Specialty: Physical Medicine and Rehabilitation
Program name: Schwab Rehabilitation Hospital and Care Network/University of Chicago Program
Program code: 340-16-22-012
State: Illinois
Address: Schwab Rehabilitation Hospital and Care

1401 S California Blvd, Chicago, IL 60608
Phone: (773) 522-5853

Fax: (773) 522-5855
Percentage of IMGs in the program: 15%
Minimum USMLE Step 1 Score Requirement:
No limits set
Minimum USMLE Step 2 Score Requirement:
No limits set
Attempts on any step: Must pass on maximum
the 2nd attempt including CS exam
CS required at time of application: No
USCE Requirement: Yes
Cut-Off time since graduation: 4 years
Program offers couple match: Yes
Visas Sponsored or accepted: No visa

Marianjoy Rehabilitation Hospital Physical Medicine and Rehabilitation Residency Program

Specialty: Physical Medicine and Rehabilitation
Program name: Marianjoy Rehabilitation
Hospital Program
Program code: 340-16-21-097
NRMP Code: 1103340A0
Program type: Community-based
State: Illinois
Address: Marianjoy Rehabilitation Hospital
        26W171 Roosevelt Rd, Wheaton, IL
60187
Phone: (630) 909-7290

Fax: (630) 909-7291
Percentage of IMGs in the program: 30%
Minimum USMLE Step 1 Score Requirement: No limits set
Minimum USMLE Step 2 Score Requirement: No limits set
Attempts on any step: No limits set
CS required at time of application: No
USCE Requirement: None
Cut-Off time since graduation: 5 years
Program offers couple match: Yes
Visas Sponsored or accepted: No visa

Rush University Medical Center Physical Medicine and Rehabilitation Residency Program

Specialty: Physical Medicine and Rehabilitation
Program name: Rush University Medical Center Program
Program code: 340-16-21-082
State: Illinois
Address: Rush University Medical Center
1725 W Harrison St, Chicago, IL 60612
Phone: (312) 942-4817
Fax: (312) 942-4234
Percentage of IMGs in the program: 30%
Minimum USMLE Step 1 Score Requirement: 210

Minimum USMLE Step 2 Score Requirement:
210
Attempts on any step: Must pass on maximum
the 2nd attempt including CS exam
CS required at time of application: Yes
USCE Requirement: Yes, 2 years
Cut-Off time since graduation: 3 years
Program offers couple match: No
Visas Sponsored or accepted: J1 visa

Kansas

University of Kansas School of Medicine Physical Medicine and Rehabilitation Residency Program

Specialty: Physical Medicine and Rehabilitation
Program name: University of Kansas School of
Medicine Program
Program code: 340-19-21-018
NRMP Code: 1208340A0
Program type: University-based
State: Kansas
Address: University of Kansas Medical Center
        3901 Rainbow Blvd, Kansas City, KS
66160

Phone: (913) 588-6777
Fax: (913) 588-6765
Percentage of IMGs in the program: 20%
Minimum USMLE Step 1 Score Requirement: No limits set
Minimum USMLE Step 2 Score Requirement: No limits set
Attempts on any step: Must pass on first attempt including CS exam
CS required at time of application: No
USCE Requirement: Yes
Cut-Off time since graduation: No limits set
Program offers couple match: Yes
Visas Sponsored or accepted: No visa

Kentucky

University of Kentucky College of Medicine Physical Medicine and Rehabilitation Residency Program

Specialty: Physical Medicine and Rehabilitation
Program name: University of Kentucky College of Medicine Program
Program code: 340-20-21-079
State: Kentucky
Address: University of Kentucky Medical Center
800 Rose St, Lexington, KY 40536-0284

Phone: (859) 257-4890
Fax: (859) 323-1123
Percentage of IMGs in the program: 50%
Minimum USMLE Step 1 Score Requirement:
No limits set
Minimum USMLE Step 2 Score Requirement:
No limits set
Attempts on any step: No limits set
CS required at time of application: No
USCE Requirement: None
Cut-Off time since graduation: No limits set
Program offers couple match: Yes
Visas Sponsored or accepted: J1 visa and H1b
visa

University of Louisville Physical Medicine and Rehabilitation Residency Program

Specialty: Physical Medicine and Rehabilitation
Program name: University of Louisville Program
Program code: 340-20-11-019
NRMP Code: 1217340A0
Program type: Community-based university
affiliated hospital
State: Kentucky
Address: University of Louisville
          220 Abraham Flexner Way, Louisville,
KY 40202
Phone: (502) 582-7465

Fax: (502) 582-7601
Percentage of IMGs in the program: 25%
Minimum USMLE Step 1 Score Requirement: No limits set
Minimum USMLE Step 2 Score Requirement: No limits set
Attempts on any step: Must pass on first attempt including CS exam
CS required at time of application: No
USCE Requirement: None
Cut-Off time since graduation: 5 years
Program offers couple match: Yes
Visas Sponsored or accepted: J1 visa

Louisiana

Louisiana State University Physical Medicine and Rehabilitation Residency Program

Specialty: Physical Medicine and Rehabilitation
Program name: Louisiana State University Program
Program code: 340-21-21-020
State: Louisiana
Address: LSU Health Science Center New Orleans

1542 Tulane Ave, New Orleans, LA 70112
Phone: (504) 568-2577
Fax: (504) 568-2127
Percentage of IMGs in the program: 0% (occasionally one)
Minimum USMLE Step 1 Score Requirement: 210
Minimum USMLE Step 2 Score Requirement: 210
Attempts on any step: Must pass on first attempt
CS required at time of application: Yes
USCE Requirement: None
Cut-Off time since graduation: 2 years
Program offers couple match: Yes
Visas Sponsored or accepted: No visa

Massachusetts

Tufts Medical Center Physical Medicine and Rehabilitation Residency Program

Specialty: Physical Medicine and Rehabilitation

Program name: Tufts Medical Center Program
Program code: 340-24-21-023
NRMP Code: 1263340A0
Program type: Community-based university affiliated hospital
State: Massachusetts
Address: Tufts Medical Center
800 Washington St, Boston, MA 02111
Phone: (617) 636-5625
Percentage of IMGs in the program: 30%
Minimum USMLE Step 1 Score Requirement: No limits set
Minimum USMLE Step 2 Score Requirement: No limits set
Attempts on any step: Must pass on first attempt including CS exam
CS required at time of application: Yes including ECFMG certificate
USCE Requirement: Yes
Cut-Off time since graduation: 3 years
Program offers couple match: Yes
Visas Sponsored or accepted: J1 visa

Michigan

William Beaumont Hospital Physical Medicine and Rehabilitation Residency Program

Specialty: Physical Medicine and Rehabilitation
Program name: William Beaumont Hospital Program
Program code: 340-25-21-076
State: Michigan
Address: William Beaumont Hospital
3601 W 13 Mile Rd, Royal Oak, MI 48073-6769
Phone: (248) 898-0161
Fax: (248) 898-3631
Percentage of IMGs in the program: 20%
Minimum USMLE Step 1 Score Requirement: No limits set
Minimum USMLE Step 2 Score Requirement: No limits set
Attempts on any step: Must pass on first attempt
CS required at time of application: Yes including ECFMG certificate
USCE Requirement: None
Cut-Off time since graduation: No limits set
Program offers couple match: Yes
Visas Sponsored or accepted: J1 visa and H1b visa

Detroit Medical Center/Wayne State University Physical Medicine and Rehabilitation Residency Program

Specialty: Physical Medicine and Rehabilitation
Program name: Detroit Medical Center/Wayne State University Program
Program code: 340-25-21-027
State: Michigan
Address: Rehabilitation Institute of Michigan
261 Mack Blvd, Detroit, MI 48201
Phone: (313) 745-9880
Fax: (313) 745-1063
Percentage of IMGs in the program: 35%
Minimum USMLE Step 1 Score Requirement: 215
Minimum USMLE Step 2 Score Requirement: 215
Attempts on any step: Must pass on first attempt including CS exam
CS required at time of application: Yes including ECFMG certificate
USCE Requirement: Yes 1 year
Cut-Off time since graduation: No limits set
Program offers couple match: No
Visas Sponsored or accepted: No visa

Wayne State University School of Medicine Physical Medicine and Rehabilitation Residency Program

Specialty: Physical Medicine and Rehabilitation
Program name: Wayne State University School of Medicine Program
Program code: 340-25-12-108
NRMP Code: 1361340C0
Program type: University-based
State: Michigan
Address: Oakwood Heritage Hospital
10000 Telegraph Rd, Taylor, MI 48180
Phone: (313) 375-7226
Fax: (313) 375-7225
Percentage of IMGs in the program: 25%
Minimum USMLE Step 1 Score Requirement: No limits set
Minimum USMLE Step 2 Score Requirement: No limits set
Attempts on any step: No limits set
CS required at time of application: Yes
USCE Requirement: None
Cut-Off time since graduation: No limits set
Program offers couple match: Yes
Visas Sponsored or accepted: No visa

Minnesota

University of Minnesota Physical Medicine and Rehabilitation Residency Program

Specialty: Physical Medicine and Rehabilitation
Program name: University of Minnesota Program
Program code: 340-26-21-028
NRMP Code: 1334340C0, 1334340A0
Program type: University-based
State: Minnesota
Address: University of Minnesota Medical Center
500 Boynton Health Service Bridge MMC 297
420 Delaware St SE, Minneapolis, MN 55455
Phone: (612) 626-4913
Fax: (612) 624-6686
Percentage of IMGs in the program: 25%
Minimum USMLE Step 1 Score Requirement: No limits set
Minimum USMLE Step 2 Score Requirement: No limits set
Attempts on any step: Prefer passing from 1st attempt
CS required at time of application: Yes including ECFMG certificate
USCE Requirement: Yes at least 1 month with LOR from PM&R preferred
Cut-Off time since graduation: 10 years
Program offers couple match: Yes
Visas Sponsored or accepted: J1 visa

Mayo Clinic College of Medicine (Rochester) Physical Medicine and Rehabilitation Residency Program

Specialty: Physical Medicine and Rehabilitation
Program name: Mayo Clinic College of Medicine (Rochester) Program
Program code: 340-26-21-030
NRMP Code: 1328340C0, 1328340A0
Program type: University-based
State: Minnesota
Address: Mayo Clinic
200 First St SW, Rochester, MN 55905
Phone: (507) 284-2946
Fax: (507) 293-1757
Percentage of IMGs in the program: 10%
Minimum USMLE Step 1 Score Requirement: No limits set
Minimum USMLE Step 2 Score Requirement: No limits set
Attempts on any step: Must pass on first attempt including CS exam
CS required at time of application: Yes including ECFMG certificate
USCE Requirement: Yes
Cut-Off time since graduation: 3 years unless clinically active
Program offers couple match: Yes
Visas Sponsored or accepted: J1 visa

Missouri

Washington University/B-JH/SLCH Consortium Physical Medicine and Rehabilitation Residency Program

Specialty: Physical Medicine and Rehabilitation
Program name: Washington University/B-JH/SLCH Consortium Program
Program code: 340-28-11-032
NRMP Code: 1353340C0, 1353340A0
Program type: University-based
State: Missouri
Address: Washington University Medical Center
4444 Forest Park Ave, St Louis, MO 63108
Phone: (314) 454-7757
Fax: (314) 454-5300
Percentage of IMGs in the program: 40%
Minimum USMLE Step 1 Score Requirement: No limits set
Minimum USMLE Step 2 Score Requirement: No limits set
Attempts on any step: No limits set

CS required at time of application: Yes
including ECFMG certificate
USCE Requirement: None
Cut-Off time since graduation: 10 years
Program offers couple match: Yes
Visas Sponsored or accepted: J1 visa

New Jersey

Rutgers New Jersey Medical School Physical Medicine and Rehabilitation Residency Program

Specialty: Physical Medicine and Rehabilitation
Program name: Rutgers New Jersey Medical
School Program (UMDNJ)
Program code: 340-33-32-034
NRMP Code: 1398340A0
Program type: Community-based university
affiliated hospital
State: New Jersey
Address: Rutgers New Jersey Medical School
        30 Bergen St, Newark, NJ 07101
Phone: (973) 972-3606
Fax: (973) 972-5148
Percentage of IMGs in the program: 15%

Minimum USMLE Step 1 Score Requirement: No limits set
Minimum USMLE Step 2 Score Requirement: No limits set
Attempts on any step: Must pass on first attempt including CS exam
CS required at time of application: No
USCE Requirement: None
Cut-Off time since graduation: No limits set
Program offers couple match: Yes
Visas Sponsored or accepted: J1 visa

New York

Kingsbrook Jewish Medical Center Physical Medicine and Rehabilitation Residency Program

Specialty: Physical Medicine and Rehabilitation
Program name: Kingsbrook Jewish Medical Center Program
Program code: 340-35-22-041
State: New York
Address: Kingsbrook Jewish Medical Center 585 Schenectady Ave, Brooklyn, NY 11203

Phone: (718) 604-5341
Fax: (718) 604-5272
Percentage of IMGs in the program: 50%
Minimum USMLE Step 1 Score Requirement: 220
Minimum USMLE Step 2 Score Requirement: 220
Attempts on any step: Must pass on maximum 2nd attempt including CS exam
CS required at time of application: Yes including ECFMG certificate
USCE Requirement: None
Cut-Off time since graduation: No limits set
Program offers couple match: Yes
Visas Sponsored or accepted: No visa

SUNY at Stony Brook Physical Medicine and Rehabilitation Residency Program

Specialty: Physical Medicine and Rehabilitation
Program name: SUNY at Stony Brook Program
Program code: 340-35-21-103
State: New York
Address: Northport VA Medical Center
            79 Middleville Rd, Northport, NY 11768
Phone: (631) 261-4400   Ext: 7198
Fax: (631) 266-6022
Percentage of IMGs in the program: 20%

Minimum USMLE Step 1 Score Requirement:
No limits set
Minimum USMLE Step 2 Score Requirement:
No limits set
Attempts on any step: Must pass on maximum
2nd attempt
CS required at time of application: Yes
including ECFMG certificate
USCE Requirement: None
Cut-Off time since graduation: No limits set but
must be clinically active
Program offers couple match: Yes
Visas Sponsored or accepted: No visa

SUNY Upstate Medical University Physical Medicine and Rehabilitation Residency Program

Specialty: Physical Medicine and Rehabilitation
Program name: SUNY Upstate Medical
University Program
Program code: 340-35-21-093
NRMP Code: 1516340A0
Program type: University-based
State: New York
Address: SUNY Upstate Medical University
         750 E Adams St, Syracuse, NY 13210-
2375
Phone: (315) 464-8672

Fax: (315) 464-8699
Percentage of IMGs in the program: 25%
Minimum USMLE Step 1 Score Requirement: 215
Minimum USMLE Step 2 Score Requirement: 215
Attempts on any step: Must pass maximum on 2nd attempt including CS exam
CS required at time of application: Yes including ECFMG certificate
USCE Requirement: None
Cut-Off time since graduation: 5 years
Program offers couple match: Yes
Visas Sponsored or accepted: J1 visa

University of Rochester Physical Medicine and Rehabilitation Program

Specialty: Physical Medicine and Rehabilitation
Program name: University of Rochester Program
Program code: 340-35-21-051
NRMP Code: 1511340C0
Program type: University-based
State: New York
Address: University of Rochester Medical Center
        601 Elmwood Ave, Rochester, NY 14642

Phone: (585) 275-3274
Fax: (585) 442-2949
Percentage of IMGs in the program: 10%
Minimum USMLE Step 1 Score Requirement: No limits set
Minimum USMLE Step 2 Score Requirement: No limits set
Attempts on any step: Must pass on first attempt
CS required at time of application: Yes including ECFMG certificate
USCE Requirement: None
Cut-Off time since graduation: No limits set
Program offers couple match: Yes
Visas Sponsored or accepted: J1 visa

SUNY Health Science Center at Brooklyn Physical Medicine and Rehabilitation Residency Program

Specialty: Physical Medicine and Rehabilitation
Program name: SUNY Health Science Center at Brooklyn Program
Program code: 340-35-21-048
NRMP Code: 1426340A0
Program type: University-based
State: New York
Address: SUNY Downstate Medical Center
        450 Clarkson Ave, Brooklyn, NY 11203
Phone: (718) 270-8128

Fax: (718) 270-8199
Percentage of IMGs in the program: 10%
Minimum USMLE Step 1 Score Requirement: 210
Minimum USMLE Step 2 Score Requirement: 210
Attempts on any step: No limits set
CS required at time of application: Yes
USCE Requirement: None
Cut-Off time since graduation: No limits set
Program offers couple match: Yes
Visas Sponsored or accepted: J1 visa and H1b visa

New York University School of Medicine Physical Medicine and Rehabilitation Residency Program

Specialty: Physical Medicine and Rehabilitation
Program name: New York University School of Medicine Program
Program code: 340-35-21-046
NRMP Code: 2978340A0
Program type: University-based
State: New York
Address: New York University Medical Center
240 E 38th St, New York, NY 10016
Phone: (212) 263-6110
Fax: (212) 263-6251
Percentage of IMGs in the program: 15%

Minimum USMLE Step 1 Score Requirement:
No limits set
Minimum USMLE Step 2 Score Requirement:
No limits set
Attempts on any step: Must pass on maximum
2nd attempt including CS exam
CS required at time of application: Yes
USCE Requirement: None
Cut-Off time since graduation: No limits set
Program offers couple match: Yes
Visas Sponsored or accepted: J1 visa

New York Medical College (Metropolitan) Physical Medicine and Rehabilitation Residency Program

Specialty: Physical Medicine and Rehabilitation
Program name: New York Medical College
(Metropolitan) Program
Program code: 340-35-21-045
State: New York
Address: New York Medical College
            40 Sunshine Cottage Rd, Valhalla, NY
10595
Phone: (914) 594-2090
Fax: (914) 594-2091
Percentage of IMGs in the program: 60%
Minimum USMLE Step 1 Score Requirement:
No limits set

Minimum USMLE Step 2 Score Requirement:
No limits set
Attempts on any step: No limits set
CS required at time of application: No
USCE Requirement: None
Cut-Off time since graduation: No limits set
Program offers couple match: No
Visas Sponsored or accepted: J1 visa and H1b visa

Albert Einstein College of Medicine Physical Medicine and Rehabilitation Residency Program

Specialty: Physical Medicine and Rehabilitation
Program name: Albert Einstein College of Medicine Program
Program code: 340-35-21-043
State: New York
Address: Montefiore Medical Center
                150 E 210th St, Bronx, NY 10467
Phone: (718) 920-2753
Fax: (718) 920-5048
Percentage of IMGs in the program: 40%
Minimum USMLE Step 1 Score Requirement:
No limits set
Minimum USMLE Step 2 Score Requirement:
No limits set
Attempts on any step: No limits set

CS required at time of application: No
USCE Requirement: None
Cut-Off time since graduation: No limits set
Program offers couple match: Yes
Visas Sponsored or accepted: J1 visa and H1b visa

NSLIJHS/Hofstra North Shore-LIJ School of Medicine Physical Medicine and Rehabilitation Residency Program

Specialty: Physical Medicine and Rehabilitation
Program name: NSLIJHS/Hofstra North Shore-LIJ School of Medicine Program
Program code: 340-35-21-042
NRMP Code: 1700340A0
Program type: University-based
State: New York
Address: North Shore-LIJ Health System
            825 Northern Blvd, Great Neck, NY 11021
Phone: (516) 465-8729
Fax: (516) 465-8723
Percentage of IMGs in the program: 50%
Minimum USMLE Step 1 Score Requirement: No limits set
Minimum USMLE Step 2 Score Requirement: No limits set

Attempts on any step: Must pass on first attempt
CS required at time of application: Yes including ECFMG certificate
USCE Requirement: None
Cut-Off time since graduation: 2 years
Program offers couple match: Yes
Visas Sponsored or accepted: J1 visa and H1b visa

Albany Medical Center Physical Medicine and Rehabilitation Residency Program

Specialty: Physical Medicine and Rehabilitation
Program name: Albany Medical Center Program
Program code: 340-35-21-035
NRMP Code: 1414340C0
Program type: University-based
State: New York
Address: Albany Medical Center
47 New Scotland Ave, Albany, NY 12208
Phone: (518) 262-6488
Fax: (518) 262-6178
Percentage of IMGs in the program: 25%
Minimum USMLE Step 1 Score Requirement: 220

Minimum USMLE Step 2 Score Requirement: 220
Attempts on any step: Must pass on first attempt
CS required at time of application: No
USCE Requirement: None
Cut-Off time since graduation: 4 years
Program offers couple match: Yes
Visas Sponsored or accepted: J1 visa

Nassau University Medical Center Physical Medicine and Rehabilitation Residency Program

Specialty: Physical Medicine and Rehabilitation
Program name: Nassau University Medical Center Program
Program code: 340-35-11-037
NRMP Code: 1448340A0
Program type: Community-based university affiliated hospital
State: New York
Address: Nassau University Medical Center
2201 Hempstead Trnpk, East Meadow, NY 11554-5400
Phone: (516) 572-6525
Fax: (516) 572-3170
Percentage of IMGs in the program: 20%
Minimum USMLE Step 1 Score Requirement: No limits set

Minimum USMLE Step 2 Score Requirement:
No limits set
Attempts on any step: No limits set
CS required at time of application: No
USCE Requirement: Yes
Cut-Off time since graduation: No limits set
Program offers couple match: Yes
Visas Sponsored or accepted: J1 visa

North Carolina

Vidant Medical Center/East Carolina University Physical Medicine and Rehabilitation Residency Program

Specialty: Physical Medicine and Rehabilitation
Program name: Vidant Medical Center/East Carolina University Program
Program code: 340-36-21-091
NRMP Code: 3057340C0
Program type: University-based
State: North Carolina
Address: Regional Rehabilitation Center
            2100 Stantonsburg Rd, Greenville, NC 27835-6028
Phone: (252) 847-7907

Fax: (252) 847-0840
Percentage of IMGs in the program: 10%
Minimum USMLE Step 1 Score Requirement: No limits set
Minimum USMLE Step 2 Score Requirement: No limits set
Attempts on any step: Must pass maximum on 2nd attempt except CS must be on 1st attempt.
CS required at time of application: Yes
USCE Requirement: Yes with at least 1 month in PM&R
Cut-Off time since graduation: 5 years
Program offers couple match: Yes
Visas Sponsored or accepted: J1 visa

Ohio

Case Western Reserve University (MetroHealth) Physical Medicine and Rehabilitation Residency Program

Specialty: Physical Medicine and Rehabilitation
Program name: Case Western Reserve University (MetroHealth) Program
Program code: 340-38-31-053
NRMP Code: 1553340C0

Program type: Community-based university affiliated hospital
State: Ohio
Address: MetroHealth Medical Center,
          4229 Pearl Rd, Cleveland, OH 44109-1998
Phone: (216) 957-3551
Fax: (216) 957-2884
Percentage of IMGs in the program: 40%
Minimum USMLE Step 1 Score Requirement: No limits set
Minimum USMLE Step 2 Score Requirement: No limits set
Attempts on any step: Must pass first attempt
CS required at time of application: Yes
USCE Requirement: 2 months
Cut-Off time since graduation: 10 years
Program offers couple match: Yes
Visas Sponsored or accepted: J1 visa and H1b visa

Pennsylvania

University of Pennsylvania Physical Medicine and Rehabilitation Residency Program

Specialty: Physical Medicine and Rehabilitation
Program name: University of Pennsylvania Program
Program code: 340-41-21-058
NRMP Code: 1628340C0, 1628340A0
Program type: University-based
State: Pennsylvania
Address: Hospital of University of Pennsylvania
1800 Lombard St, Philadelphia, PA 19146
Phone: (215) 893-2676
Fax: (215) 893-2686
Percentage of IMGs in the program: 15%
Minimum USMLE Step 1 Score Requirement: No limits set
Minimum USMLE Step 2 Score Requirement: No limits set
Attempts on any step: No limits set
CS required at time of application: Yes
USCE Requirement: None
Cut-Off time since graduation: No limits set
Program offers couple match: Yes
Visas Sponsored or accepted: No visa

Thomas Jefferson University Physical Medicine and Rehabilitation Residency Program

Specialty: Physical Medicine and Rehabilitation
Program name: Thomas Jefferson University Program
Program code: 340-41-21-057
NRMP Code: 1630340A0
Program type: University-based
State: Pennsylvania
Address: Thomas Jefferson University Hospital
25 S 9th St, Philadelphia, PA 19107
Phone: (215) 955-6585
Fax: (215) 955-2311
Percentage of IMGs in the program: 10%
Minimum USMLE Step 1 Score Requirement: No limits set
Minimum USMLE Step 2 Score Requirement: No limits set
Attempts on any step: Must pass maximum on 2nd attempt including CS exam
CS required at time of application: Yes including ECFMG certificate
USCE Requirement: Yes 1 month
Cut-Off time since graduation: 10 years
Program offers couple match: Yes
Visas Sponsored or accepted: J1 visa and H1b visa

Texas

University of Texas at Houston Physical Medicine and Rehabilitation Residency Program

Specialty: Physical Medicine and Rehabilitation
Program name: University of Texas at Houston Program
Program code: 340-48-21-101
NRMP Code: 2923340A0
Program type: Community-based university affiliated hospital
State: Texas
Address: University of Texas Health Science Center Houston
    1333 Moursund St, Houston, TX 77030-3405
Phone: (713) 799-5033
Fax: (713) 797-5982
Percentage of IMGs in the program: 20%
Minimum USMLE Step 1 Score Requirement: No limits set
Minimum USMLE Step 2 Score Requirement: No limits set

Attempts on any step: Must pass on first attempt
CS required at time of application: Yes including ECFMG certificate
USCE Requirement: Yes
Cut-Off time since graduation: No limits set
Program offers couple match: Yes
Visas Sponsored or accepted: J1 visa

University of Texas Health Science Center at San Antonio Physical Medicine and Rehabilitation Residency Program

Specialty: Physical Medicine and Rehabilitation
Program name: University of Texas Health Science Center at San Antonio Program
Program code: 340-48-21-067
NRMP Code: 1722340C0
Program type: University-based
State: Texas
Address: University of Texas Health Science Center San Antonio
            7703 Floyd Curl Dr, San Antonio, TX 78229-3900
Phone: (210) 567-5359
Fax: (210) 567-5354
Percentage of IMGs in the program: 10%
Minimum USMLE Step 1 Score Requirement: No limits set

Minimum USMLE Step 2 Score Requirement: No limits set

Attempts on any step: Maximum of 5 attempts on any step including CS exam

CS required at time of application: Yes including ECFMG certificate

USCE Requirement: Yes 1month

Cut-Off time since graduation: No limits set

Program offers couple match: Yes

Visas Sponsored or accepted: J1 visa

Baylor College of Medicine Physical Medicine and Rehabilitation Residency Program

Specialty: Physical Medicine and Rehabilitation

Program name: Baylor College of Medicine Program

Program code: 340-48-21-066

NRMP Code: 1716340A0

Program type: University-based

State: Texas

Address: Baylor College of Medicine
        1331 Moursund St, Houston, TX 77030-3405

Phone: (713) 799-5033

Fax: (713) 797-5982

Percentage of IMGs in the program: 80%

Minimum USMLE Step 1 Score Requirement: No limits set

Minimum USMLE Step 2 Score Requirement:
No limits set
Attempts on any step: No limits set
CS required at time of application: Yes
including ECFMG certificate
USCE Requirement: Yes
Cut-Off time since graduation: No limits set
Program offers couple match: Yes
Visas Sponsored or accepted: J1 visa

University of Texas Southwestern Medical School Physical Medicine and Rehabilitation Residency Program

Specialty: Physical Medicine and Rehabilitation
Program name: University of Texas
Southwestern Medical School Program
Program code: 340-48-21-065
NRMP Code: 2835340A0
Program type: Community-based university
affiliated hospital
State: Texas
Address: University of Texas Southwestern
Medical Center
        5323 Harry Hines Blvd, Dallas, TX
75390-9055
Phone: (214) 648-8826

Fax: (214) 648-9207
Percentage of IMGs in the program: 30%
Minimum USMLE Step 1 Score Requirement: No limits set
Minimum USMLE Step 2 Score Requirement: No limits set
Attempts on any step: No limits set
CS required at time of application: No
USCE Requirement: None
Cut-Off time since graduation: 10 years
Program offers couple match: Yes
Visas Sponsored or accepted: J1 visa

University of Texas Southwestern Medical School (Austin) Physical Medicine and Rehabilitation Residency Program

Specialty: Physical Medicine and Rehabilitation
Program name: University of Texas Southwestern Medical School (Austin) Program
Program code: 340-48-00-109
State: Texas
Address: University of Texas Southwestern Medical School Austin
        1400 North I-35, Austin, TX 78701
Phone: (512) 324-8235
Fax: (512) 324-8223
Percentage of IMGs in the program: 10%

Minimum USMLE Step 1 Score Requirement:
No limits set
Minimum USMLE Step 2 Score Requirement:
No limits set
Attempts on any step: No limits set
CS required at time of application: No
USCE Requirement: None
Cut-Off time since graduation: 10 years
Program offers couple match: Yes
Visas Sponsored or accepted: J1 visa

Utah

University of Utah Physical Medicine and Rehabilitation Residency Program

Specialty: Physical Medicine and Rehabilitation
Program name: University of Utah Program
Program code: 340-49-21-068
NRMP Code: 1732340C0, 1732340A0
Program type: University-based
State: Utah
Address: University of Utah Medical Center
            30 N 1900 E, Salt Lake City, UT 84132-2119

Phone: (801) 585-2589
Fax: (801) 587-7287
Percentage of IMGs in the program: 20%
Minimum USMLE Step 1 Score Requirement:
No limits set
Minimum USMLE Step 2 Score Requirement:
No limits set
Attempts on any step: Must pass maximum on
2nd attempt including CS exam
CS required at time of application: Yes
including ECFMG certificate
USCE Requirement: None
Cut-Off time since graduation: No limits set
Program offers couple match: Yes
Visas Sponsored or accepted: J1 visa

Virginia

Eastern Virginia Medical School Physical Medicine and Rehabilitation Residency Program

Specialty: Physical Medicine and Rehabilitation
Program name: Eastern Virginia Medical School
Program
Program code: 340-51-21-081

NRMP Code: 2980340A0
Program type: Community-based university affiliated hospital
State: Virginia
Address: Eastern Virginia Medical School
            721 Fairfax Ave, Norfolk, VA 23507-1912
Phone: (757) 446-5915
Fax: (757) 446-5969
Percentage of IMGs in the program: 15%
Minimum USMLE Step 1 Score Requirement: No limits set
Minimum USMLE Step 2 Score Requirement: No limits set
Attempts on any step: No limits set
CS required at time of application: Yes including ECFMG certificate
USCE Requirement: None
Cut-Off time since graduation: No limits set
Program offers couple match: No
Visas Sponsored or accepted: No visa

Virginia Commonwealth University Health System Physical Medicine and Rehabilitation Residency Program

Specialty: Physical Medicine and Rehabilitation
Program name: Virginia Commonwealth University Health System Program

Program code: 340-51-21-069
State: Virginia
Address: Virginia Commonwealth University
Health System
North Hosp 1st Fl Box 980661
1300 E Marshall St
Richmond, VA 23298
Phone: (804) 828-4233
Fax: (804) 828-5074
Percentage of IMGs in the program: 10%
Minimum USMLE Step 1 Score Requirement:
No limits set
Minimum USMLE Step 2 Score Requirement:
No limits set
Attempts on any step: No limits set
CS required at time of application: Yes
including ECFMG certificate
USCE Requirement: Yes 12 months including a
US LOR from PM&R
Cut-Off time since graduation: 4 years
Program offers couple match: Yes
Visas Sponsored or accepted: J1 visa

Washington

University of Washington Physical Medicine and Rehabilitation Residency Program

Specialty: Physical Medicine and Rehabilitation
Program name: University of Washington Program
Program code: 340-54-21-070
NRMP Code: 1918340C0, 1918340A0
Program type: University-based
State: Washington
Address: University of Washington School of Medicine
                1959 NE Pacific St, Seattle, WA 98195-6490
Phone: (206) 685-0936
Fax: (206) 616-3908
Percentage of IMGs in the program: 0% (Occasional one)
Minimum USMLE Step 1 Score Requirement: 200
Minimum USMLE Step 2 Score Requirement: 210
Attempts on any step: Must pass on first attempt including CS exam
CS required at time of application: Yes including ECFMG certificate
USCE Requirement: Yes 12 months including PM&R rotation
Cut-Off time since graduation: No limits set
Program offers couple match: Yes

Visas Sponsored or accepted: J1 visa

Wisconsin

Medical College of Wisconsin Affiliated Hospitals Physical Medicine and Rehabilitation Residency Program

Specialty: Physical Medicine and Rehabilitation
Program name: Medical College of Wisconsin Affiliated Hospitals Program
NRMP Code: 1784340A0
Program type: University-based
State: Wisconsin
Address: Froedtert Memorial Lutheran Hospital
            9200 W Wisconsin Ave, Milwaukee, WI 53226
Phone: (414) 805-9770
Fax: (414) 955-0104
Percentage of IMGs in the program: 0% (Occasional one)
Minimum USMLE Step 1 Score Requirement: No limits set
Minimum USMLE Step 2 Score Requirement: No limits set

Attempts on any step: Must pass on first attempt
CS required at time of application: No
USCE Requirement: Yes including PM&R rotation with US LOR
Cut-Off time since graduation: 2 years
Program offers couple match: Yes
Visas Sponsored or accepted: No visa

Table of Contents

Please take 1 minute to write a review and rate our book on Amazon. We wish you a successful match. Thank you for buying our book.

If you have any questions please email us at applicantguide@yahoo.com

IMG Guide
&
Applicant Guide

www.imgguide.com
www.applicantguide.com